8115  c.1

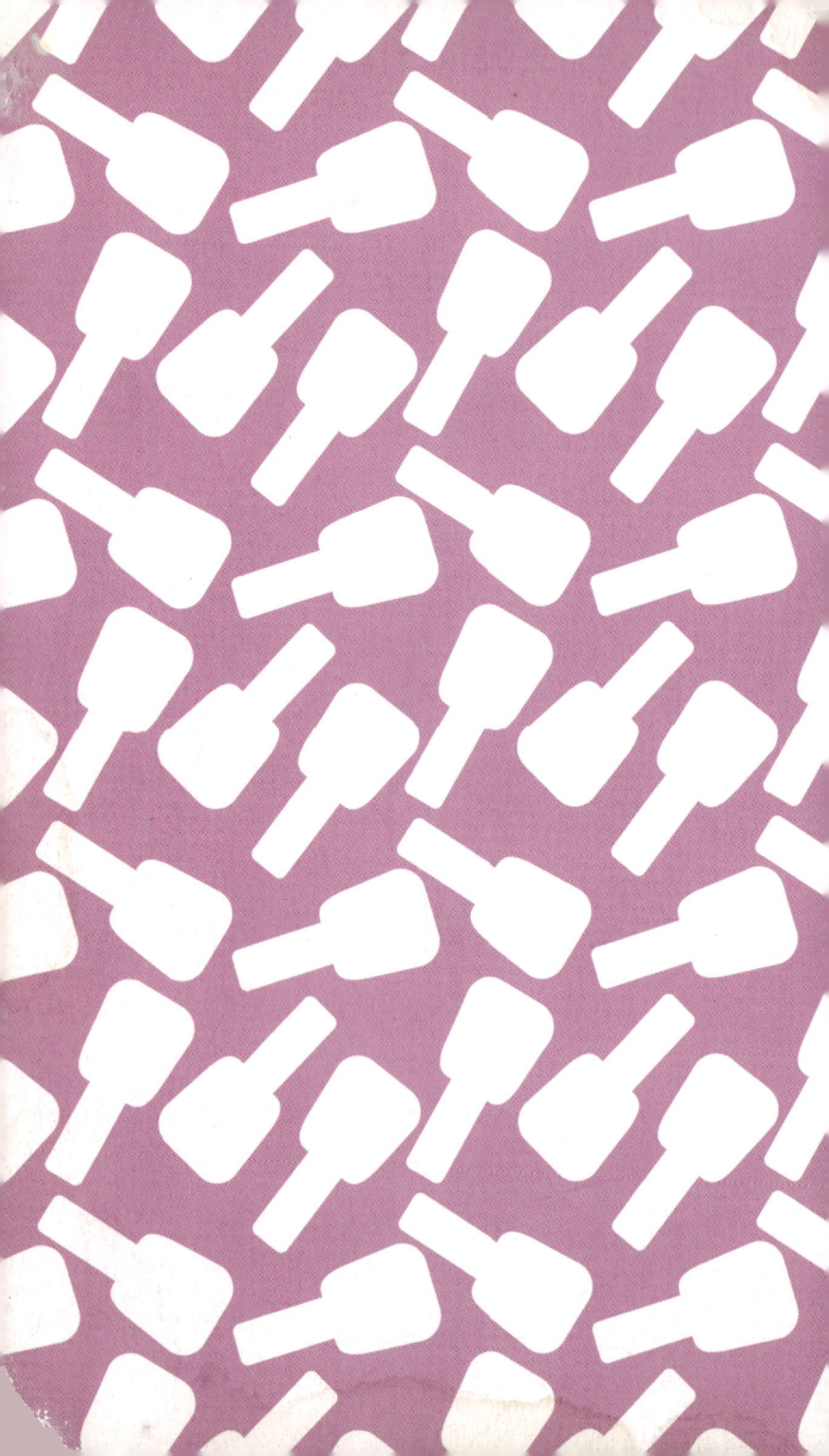

# Nail Art

Your hands say a lot about you; they are the main characters in thousands of things you do every day, and they reflect your personality. Having beautiful, cared-for hands and nails means possessing a very effective and glamorous means of expression.

With nail art, you can give a personal and fashionable touch to your nails, making them undisputed key players in creating your look. Explore colors and creativity, discover the latest techniques of this fascinating art, follow our practical tips for a perfect manicure and for the health of your nails, and be inspired by our suggestions to give your hands a unique and different look every time, depending on the occasion and your mood.

Sharpen your talons and . . . unleash your imagination!

# Perfect hands . . . perfect manicure!

### Step 1: Cleanliness

Get a bowl of warm water, hand soap, and a nail brush.

Let your hands soak for 5 minutes; then run the brush over the soap and gently scrub the tips of your fingers to clean them of all impurities. Rinse with warm water and dry your hands with a clean towel.

### Step 2: Hydration

Hydrate hands and nails with an emollient cream, letting it stand for a few minutes. If you have hands with very dry and damaged skin, you can use traditional remedies that are very effective, such as applying almond oil to your hands every night before going to bed and wearing cotton gloves throughout the night.

When your hands are soft and well-hydrated, it will be much easier to perform the manicure.

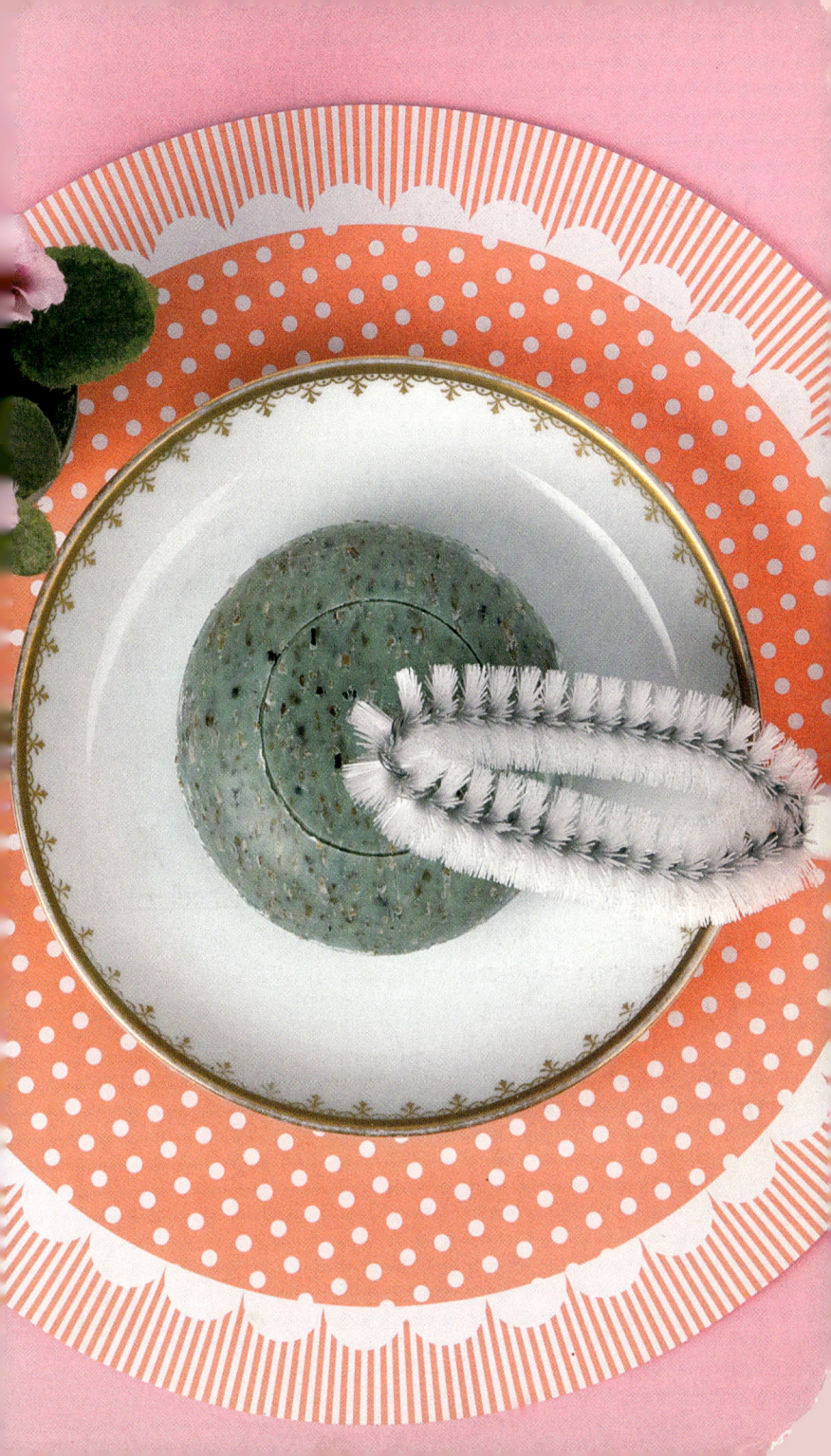

## Step 3: Care

Get nail scissors, nail clippers, and an orangewood stick cuticle pusher. Carefully remove any hardened cuticles with the clippers and adjust the shape and length of the nails with scissors.

Dip the orangewood stick (or plastic stick with a rubberized tip) in almond oil and push the cuticles to the base of the nail. Gently eliminate any remaining cuticle with the tip of the stick and rinse your hands.

## Step 4: Finishing

With totally dry hands, refine the shape of the nail with an emery board by always moving it in the same direction—from the corner towards the center—and never back and forth, so as not to damage the nail.

Give one last touch to level out the surface of the nail by using a smoothing buffer, lightly rubbing the edges: you will achieve a smooth, glossy base, which is perfect as a foundation for starting your nail art.

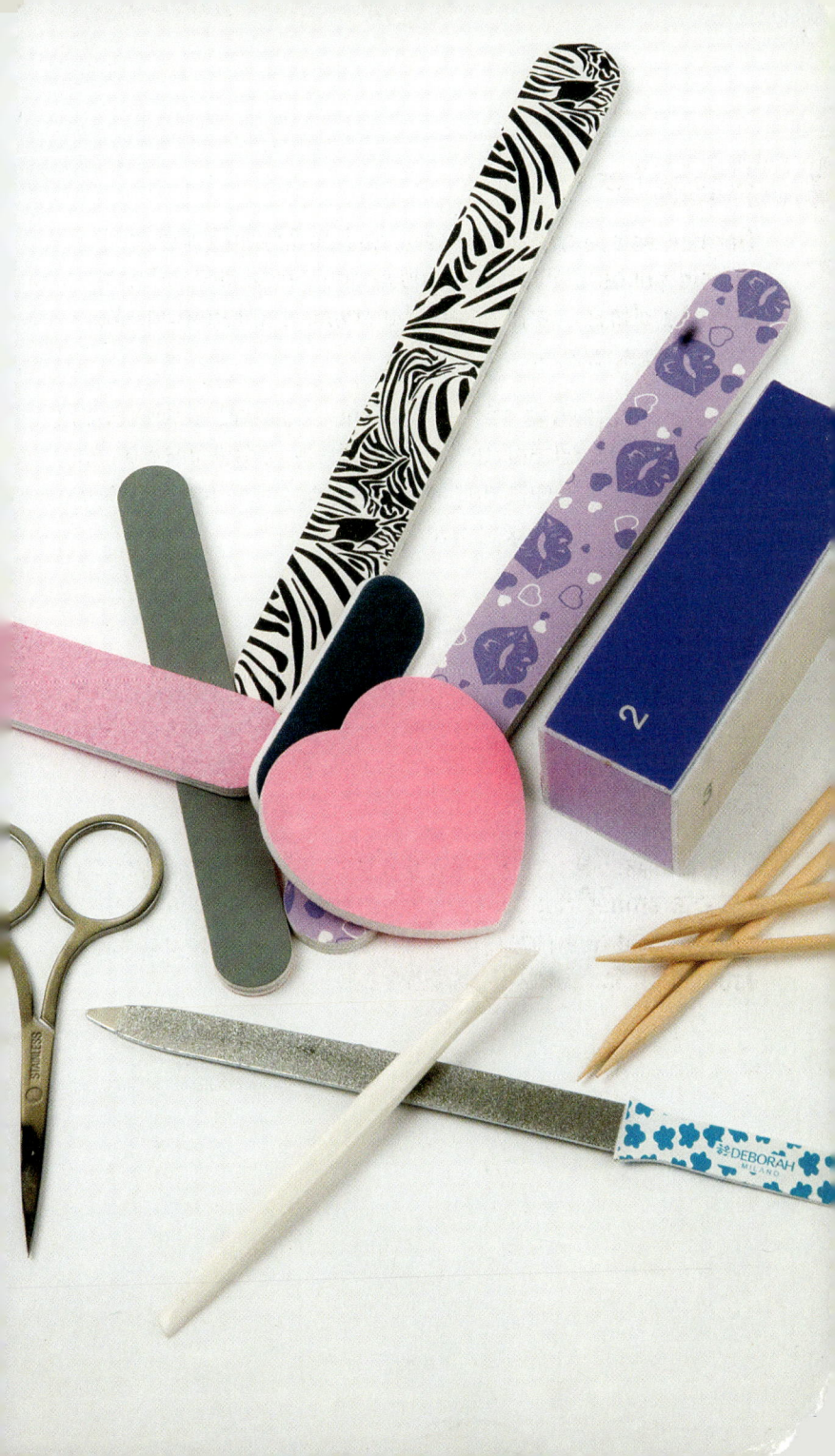

# What you will need:

The basic tools to make your nails into true masterpieces are:

- ❋ Base coat: to protect and whiten the nail; facilitates the nail polish application.

- ❋ Colored nail polish of your choice: gel, matte, glitter, shimmer . . . the varieties are many and colorful! Remember to apply the polish by always starting with a central line and then carefully drawing lines on either side, without going outside the edges of the nail.

- ❋ Top coat: clear setting nail polish, essential to giving your work some shine, as well as to refine it and protect it.

- ❋ Aluminum foil (you only need a small piece) or a cap to retain any spills: they will serve as a palette.

- ❋ Fake nails with adhesive: they are easier to decorate!

- ❋ Manicure scissors: these give fake nails the length and shape you want.

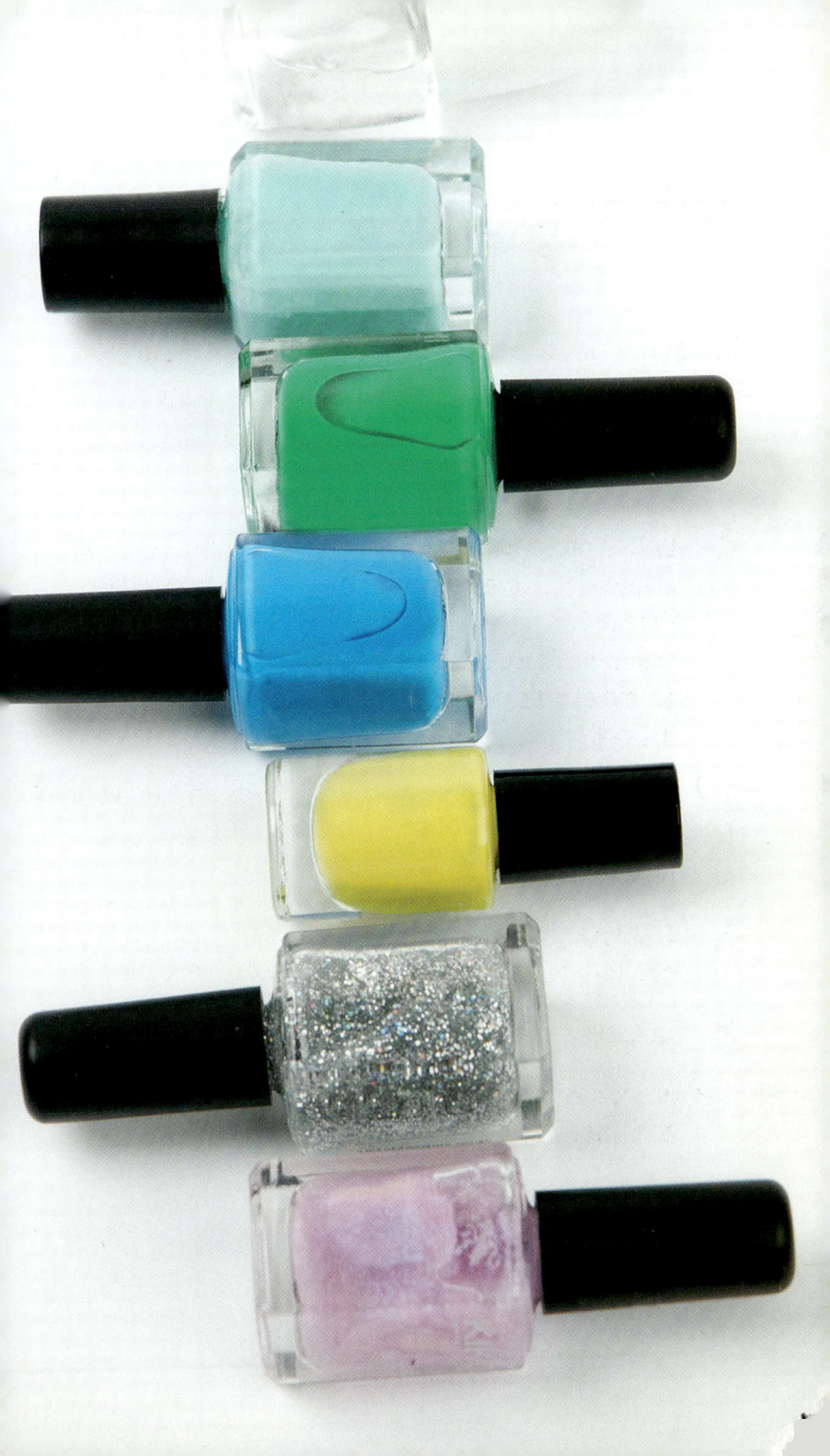

✳ Nail art brushes in fine and medium sizes: use these to paint your creations.

✳ Dotter: a stick with two points, one small and one big—this is crucial for decorations. If you do not have one on hand, and the designs that you have chosen do not require maximum precision, you can substitute the rubber tip of an open bobby pin.

✳ Tweezers: these are essential for applying your decorations.

✳ Decorations: rhinestones, feathers, glitter, and nail tattoos and appliqués of your choice will make your nails look exquisite!

## Project Legend

**WHAT'S NECESSARY:**

Tools　　Base　　Nail art　　Other　　Finishing

**DEGREE OF DIFFICULTY:**

✳ Easy　　✳✳ Medium　　✳✳✳ Expert

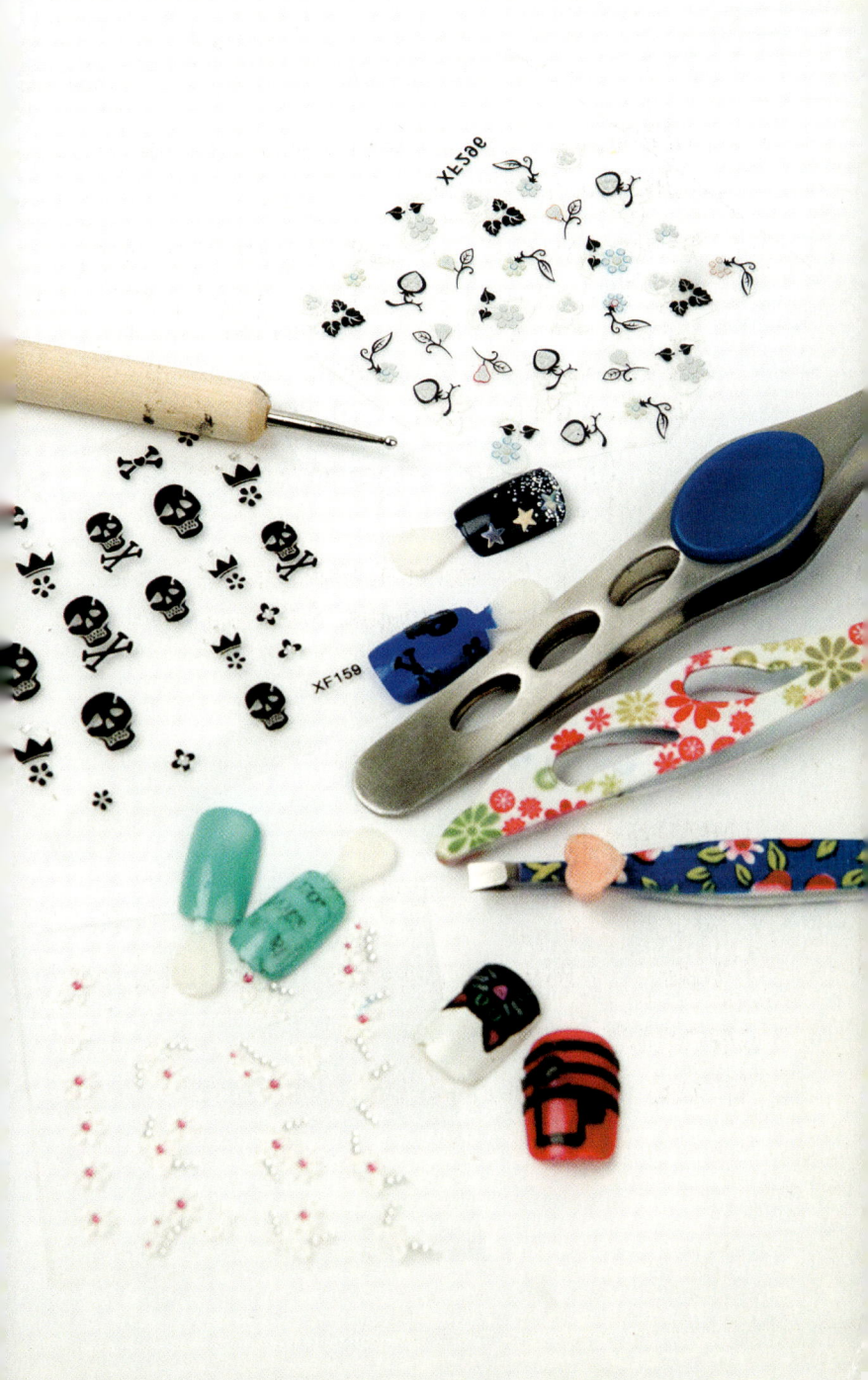

Difficulty ✻

# Polka dots!
## *A fun and retro look*

dotter    base coat    red and white nail polish    aluminum foil    top coat

1. Spread the base coat on the nail and let dry.

2. Apply the red nail polish by starting with a center line and filling in the nail with two brush strokes on either side; avoid going outside the edges. Let dry and apply another coat.

3. Put a few drops of white nail polish on the piece of aluminum foil; then dip the tip of the dotter into the nail polish and make polka dots on the nail. Let them dry thoroughly, so that when you apply the top coat your artwork does not come off.

4. Give the nails shine and protection with an application of top coat.

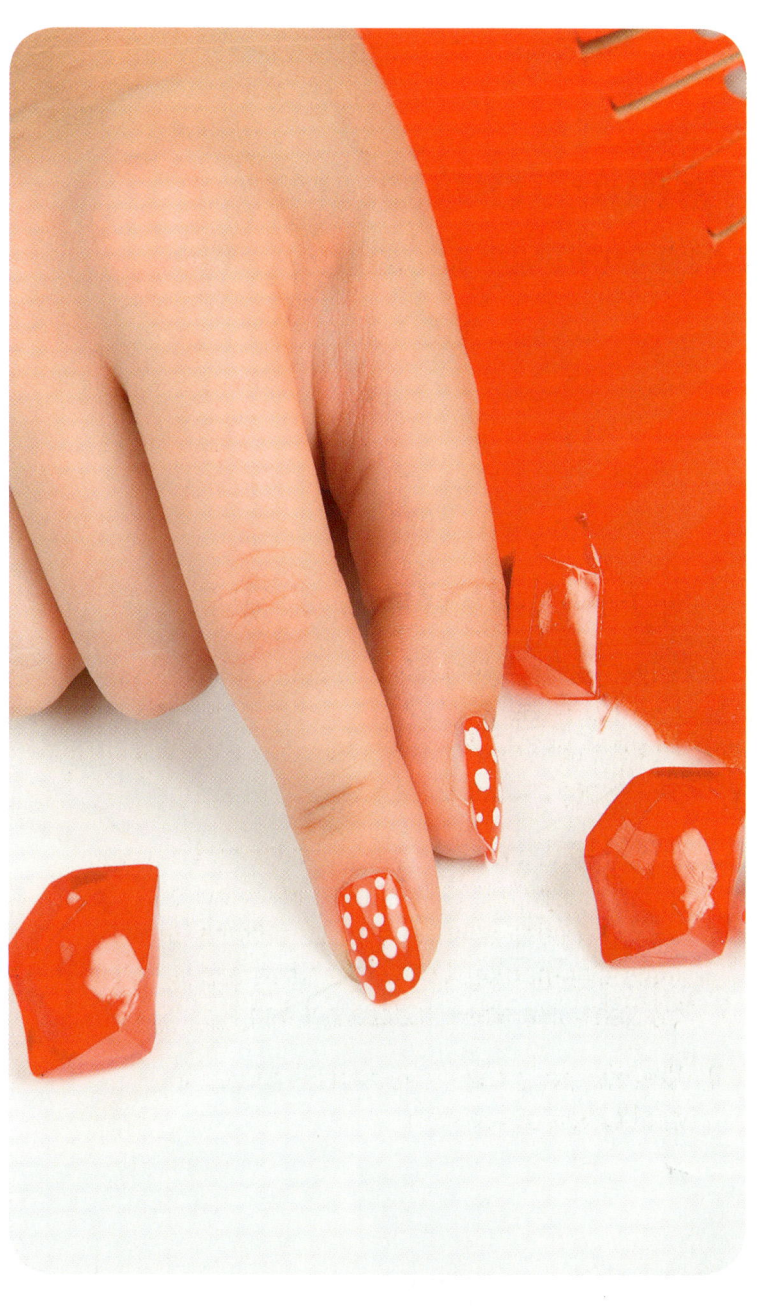

Difficulty ✸✸

# Musical notes
## *A symphony at your fingertips*

 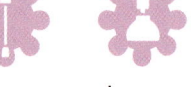   

fine brush and dotter | base coat | fuchsia and black nail polish | adhesive tape for nail art | top coat

1. Apply two coats of fuchsia nail polish over the transparent base coat. Let them dry well.

2. Pour a few drops of black nail polish on the aluminum foil; with the fine brush and a steady hand, draw a musical staff (practice drawing these on a sheet of paper). To make precise lines, use strips of adhesive tape for nail art as a guide. Let dry thoroughly.

3. Choose the musical notes that most agree with your mood and, with the fine-tipped brush and dotter, draw them on the staff. Let dry.

4. Give your decoration some shine with the top coat.

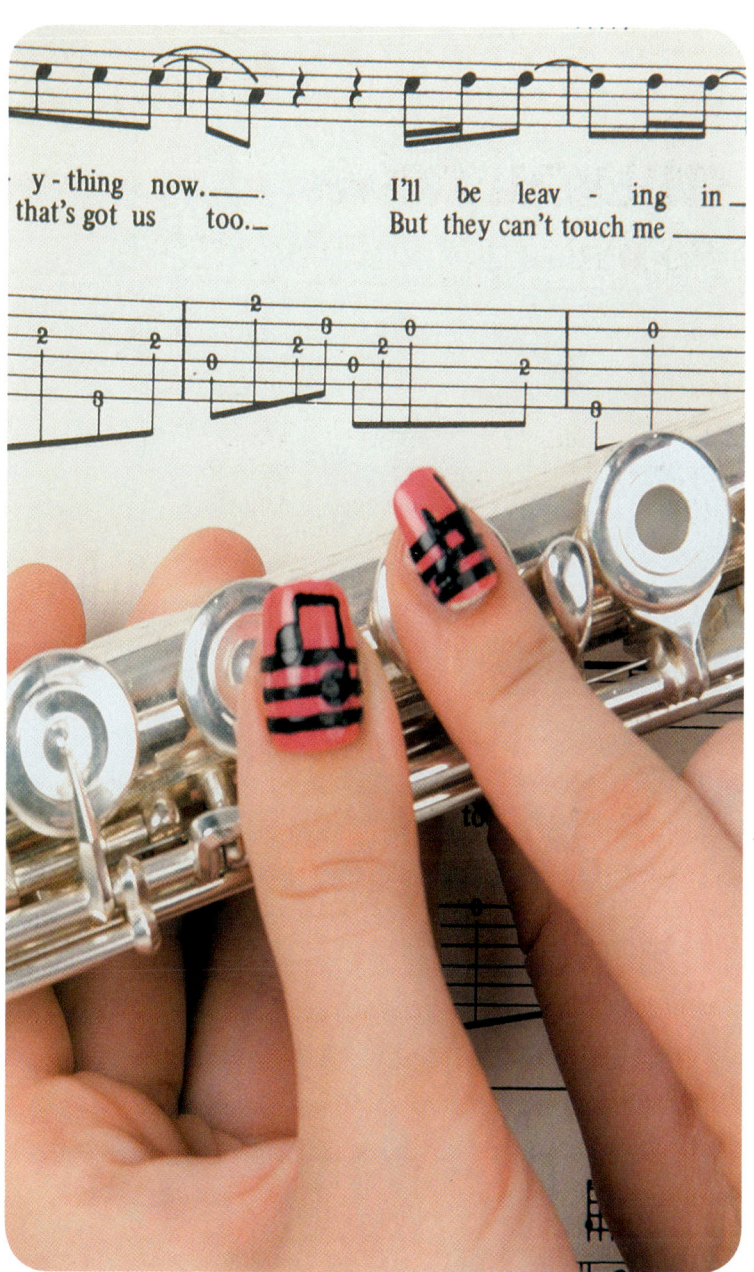

Difficulty ✽✽✽

# Owls
## *For nocturnal spirits*

fine brush and dotter • base coat • electric blue, black, yellow, brown, white, and orange nail polish • top coat

1. Start with two coats of electric blue nail polish over the base coat. Let the nail polish dry thoroughly after each application.

2. With the brush and the dotter, draw the outline of a brown owl. Trace a lighter semicircle (mix together some brown and white nail polish) for the stomach.

3. With the dotter, make yellow circles for the eyes. With the brush and black nail polish, trace the dot of the pupils; with the orange polish, draw the beak.

4. Complete with an application of top coat.

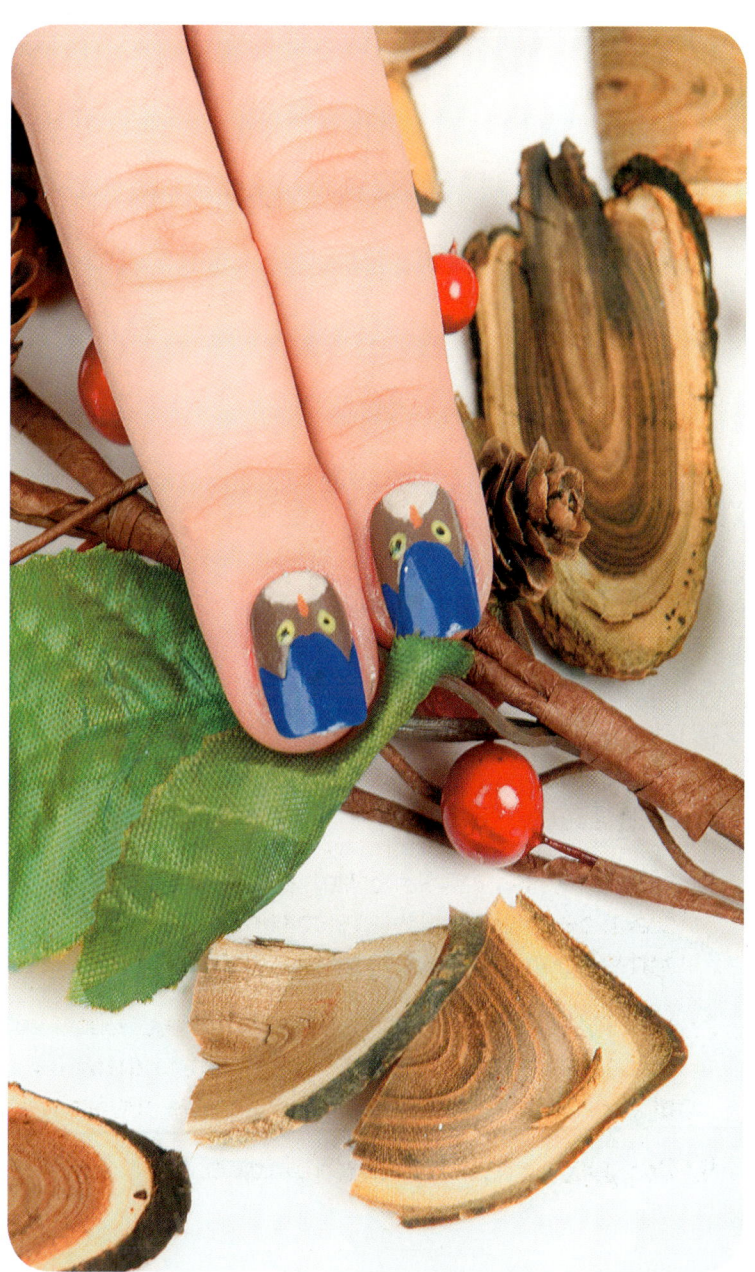

Difficulty ✸✸✸

# Cute pandas
## Cuddles and caresses

 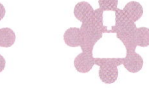   

fine brush and dotter | base coat | turquoise, white, and black nail polish | aluminum foil | top coat

1. On top of a dry base coat, apply two coats of turquoise nail polish.

2. Draw a white semicircle on the lower part of the nail and let dry.

3. Pour a small amount of black nail polish on the aluminum foil; then dip the dotter into the polish and draw two ovals for the ears, followed by two circles for the eyes and one for the nose. With the white polish and the cleaned dotter make a smaller circle inside the two black eye circles, and an even smaller black circle inside the eye circles for the pupils.

4. Finish with an application of the top coat.

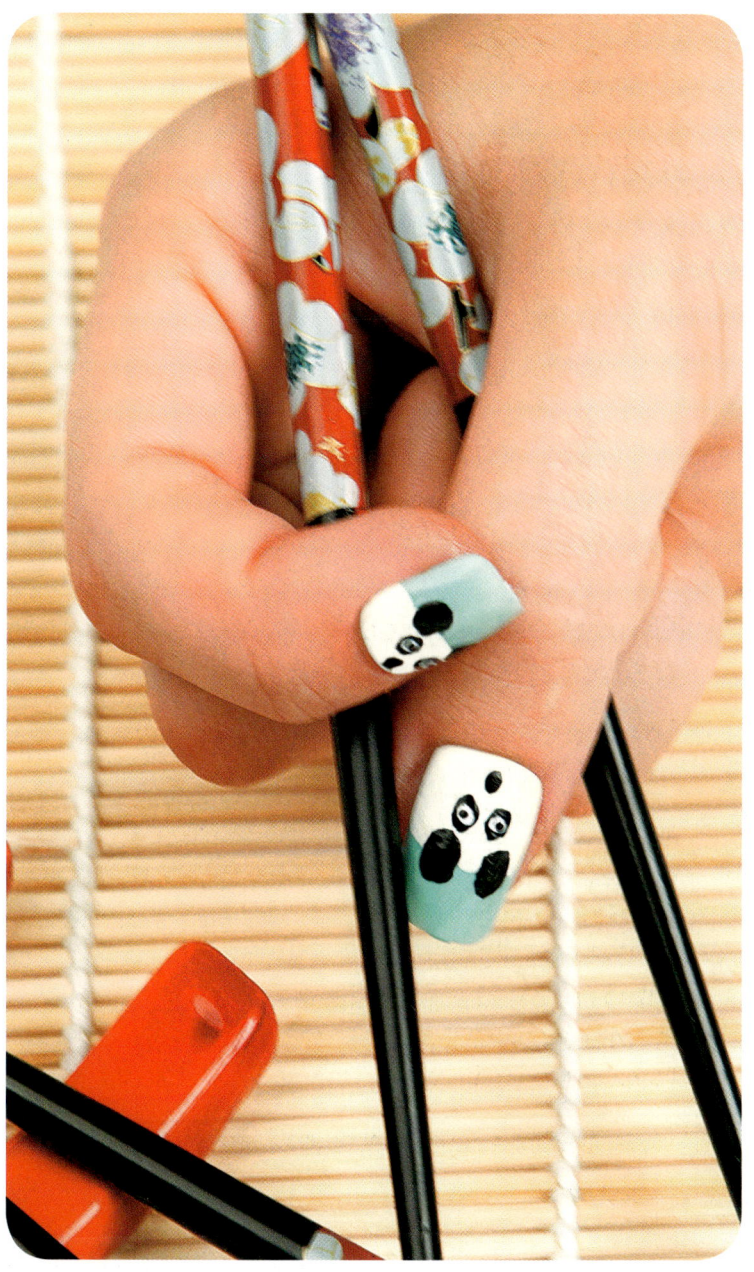

Difficulty ✻

# Clouds
## *Touch the sky with just a finger*

fine brush and dotter | base coat | light blue and white nail polish | aluminum foil | top coat

1. On a perfectly dry base coat, apply two coats of light blue nail polish and let dry thoroughly.

2. Pour a few drops of white nail polish on the aluminum foil and dip the dotter in the polish.

3. With a steady hand and using the fine brush, draw clouds scattered across the nail.

4. Let dry well and apply a top coat to finish.

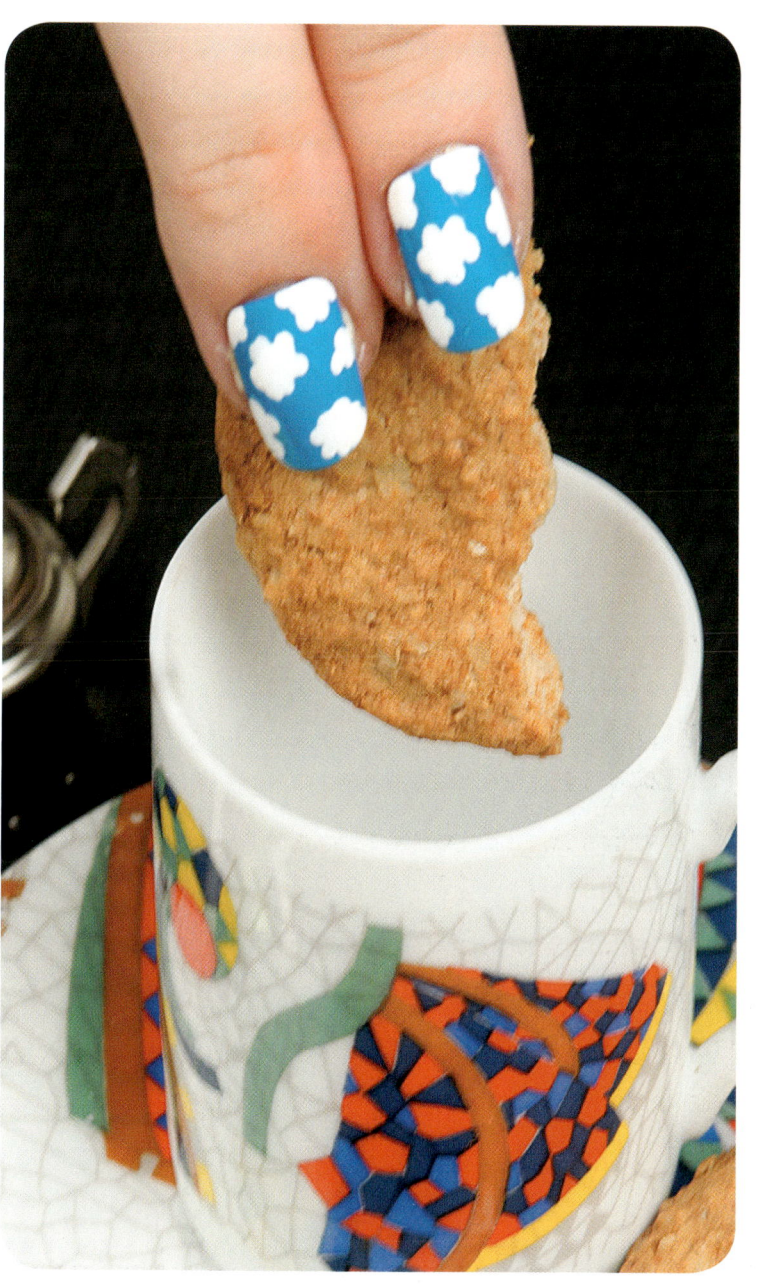

Difficulty ✸✸

# Daily News
## Special edition

scissors and tweezers

base coat

turquoise nail polish

news-paper, alcohol

top coat

1. After applying the base coat, make two applications of your favorite color nail polish. It should be bright enough to contrast with the black ink.

2. Using a newspaper, cut out the words of your choice to form a message, or you can just use a piece of a page (make sure that there is no type on the other side).

3. Using the tweezers, lightly dip your inked words into the alcohol; then place the piece of newspaper on the nail and hold for a few seconds. Gently remove the paper.

4. Check that the ink transferred well onto the fingernail; secure it with an application of top coat.

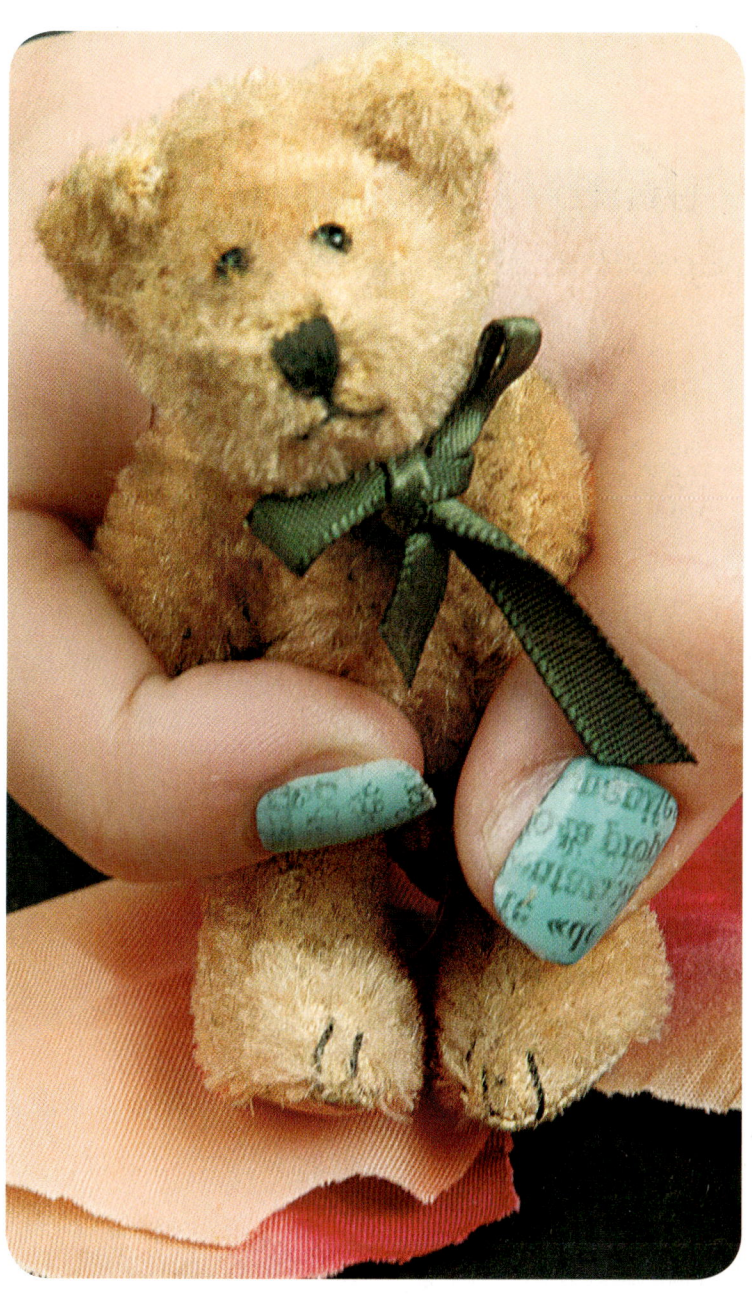

Difficulty ✸✸

# Longing for summer
## *Strawberry or watermelon?*

| fine brush and dotter | base coat | red, black, white, green, and dark green nail polish | | top coat |

1. On top of the base coat, apply two coats of red nail polish and let dry.

2. For the strawberry: with green nail polish and the brush, make a scalloped line at the tip of the nail. Finish it by adding seeds made by dipping the dotter in the black nail polish.

3. For the watermelon: with the brush, draw a green strip at the base of the nail, followed by dark green stripes. Draw a thin white stripe above the green one. The seeds are blacks dots made with the dotter.

4. Apply the top coat.

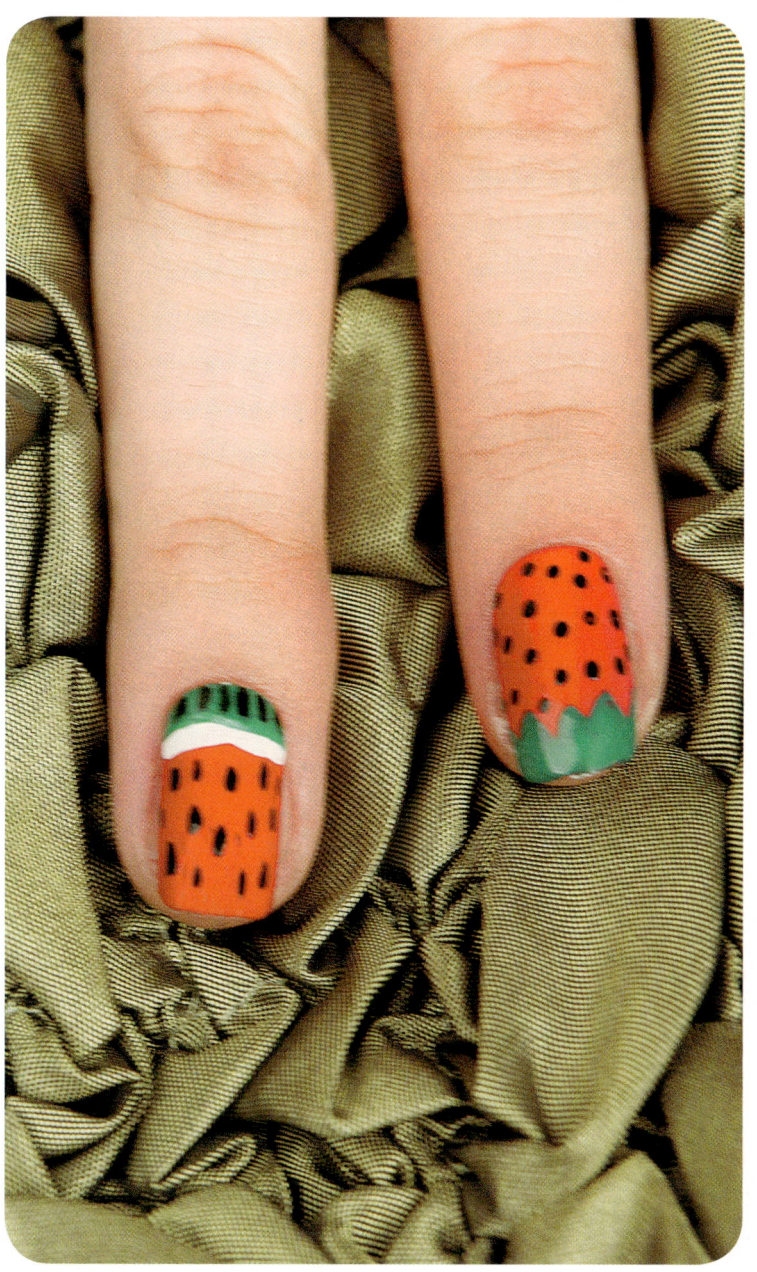

Difficulty ✱

# Ladybug
## Luck at your fingertips

medium brush and dotter | base coat | red, white, and black nail polish | aluminum foil | top coat

1. Apply the base coat and let it dry thoroughly; then apply two coats of red nail polish. Let dry.

2. Make the ladybug's head by using the medium brush to make a horizontal line of black nail polish on the tip of the nail. Draw a vertical line at the center of the nail and draw the dots with the dotter on the inside of each of the two halves of the nail.

3. With a clean dotter, draw two white dots for eyes on the black line. Let dry; then draw the pupils of the eyes using the dotter, cleaned and tinted with a few drops of black nail polish.

4. Finish off with one application of top coat.

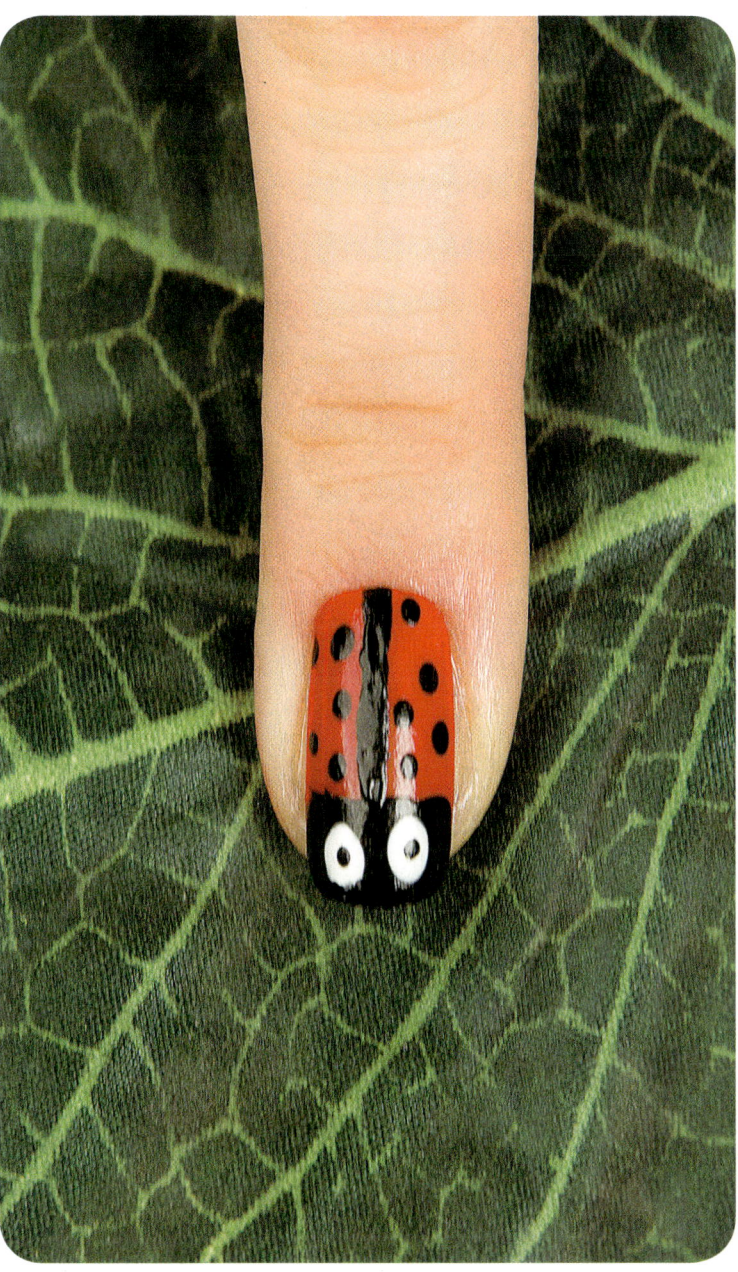

Difficulty ❄

# Snowflake
## *Surprises under your gloves*

fine brush and dotter | base coat | blue and matte white nail polish | | top coat

---

1. After applying the base coat, make two applications of blue nail polish.

2. With the fine brush, take a very small amount of white nail polish directly from the brush in the nail polish and draw different lines, crossing them to create the half-snowflake vertically on each nail.

3. Finish with the dotter, drawing dots at the end of each white line; you can make whole or half-snowflakes of different sizes.

4. Finish with a top coat, and you will have beautiful snowflakes decorating your nails!

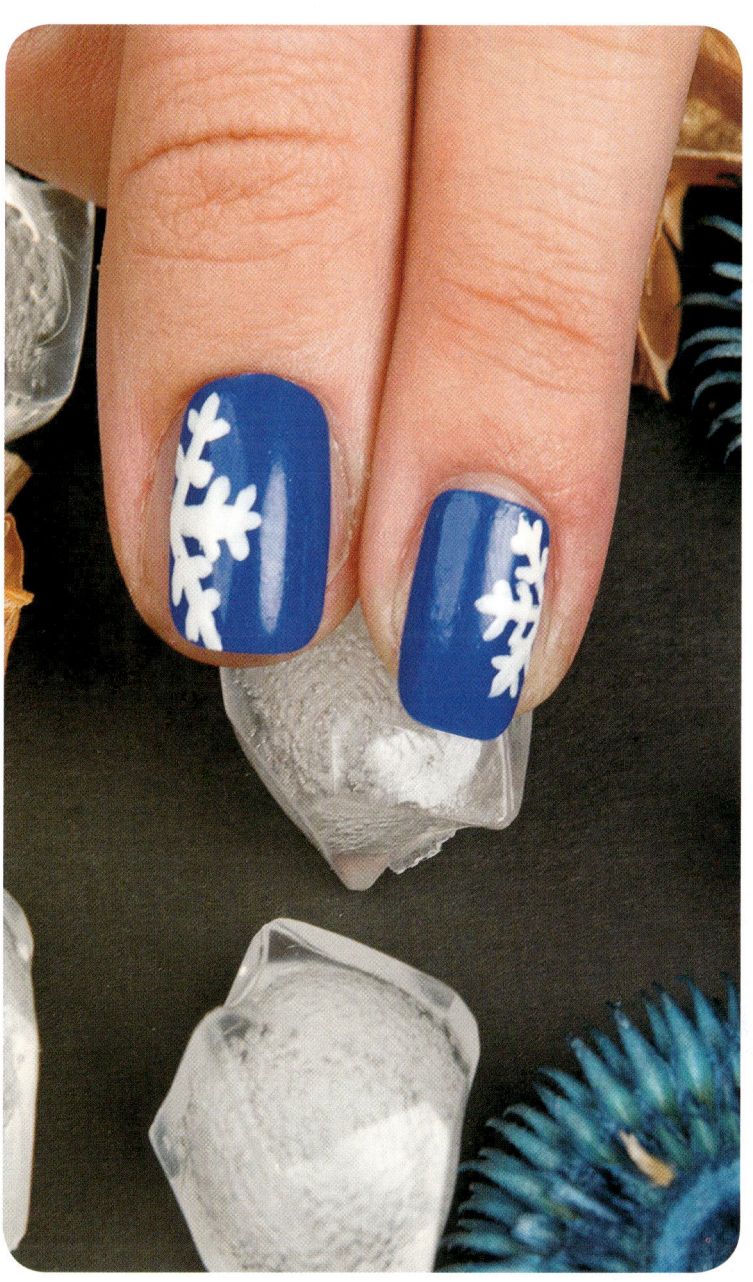

Difficulty ✸✸✸

# Moon and stars
## *A magical night*

tweezers · base coat · dark blue nail polish · glitter and moon and star appliqués · top coat

1. Apply two coats of dark blue nail polish over a perfectly dry base coat.

2. When the nail polish is nearly dry, brighten up your nails with the glitter. Use the appliqués after the nail polish is completely dry.

3. Using your tweezers, take the moon- and star-shaped appliqués and place them gently on the nail, in a design of your choice.

4. Seal everything in place with the top coat.

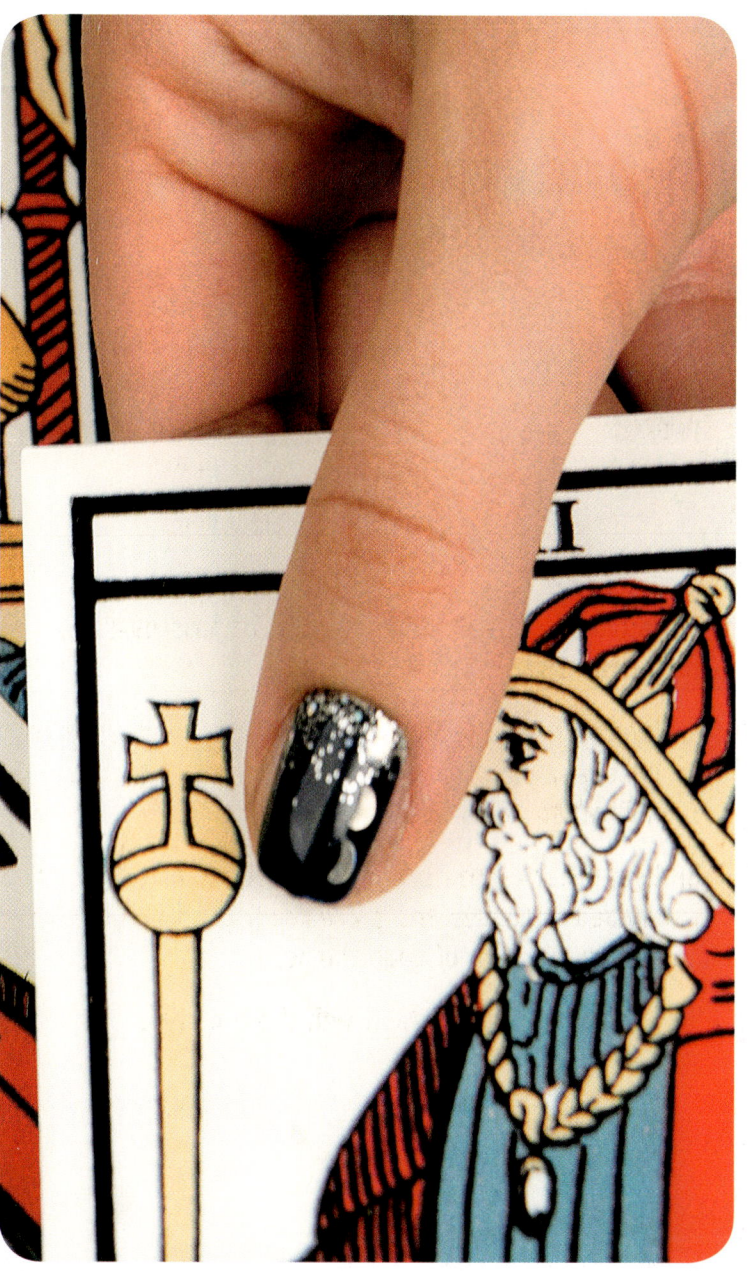

Difficulty ❋ ❋

# Tuxedo
## *This dark suit is delightful!*

fine brush and dotter | base coat | white and black nail polish | | top coat

1. Apply a base coat on the nail and let dry.

2. Apply two coats of black nail polish over the base coat. When completely dry, draw a white V for the shirt, using the fine brush.

3. Dip the dotter in the black nail polish and make a row of buttons; then, with the fine brush, draw the bow tie.

4. One application of top coat, and you're ready for your nails to enjoy a gala evening!

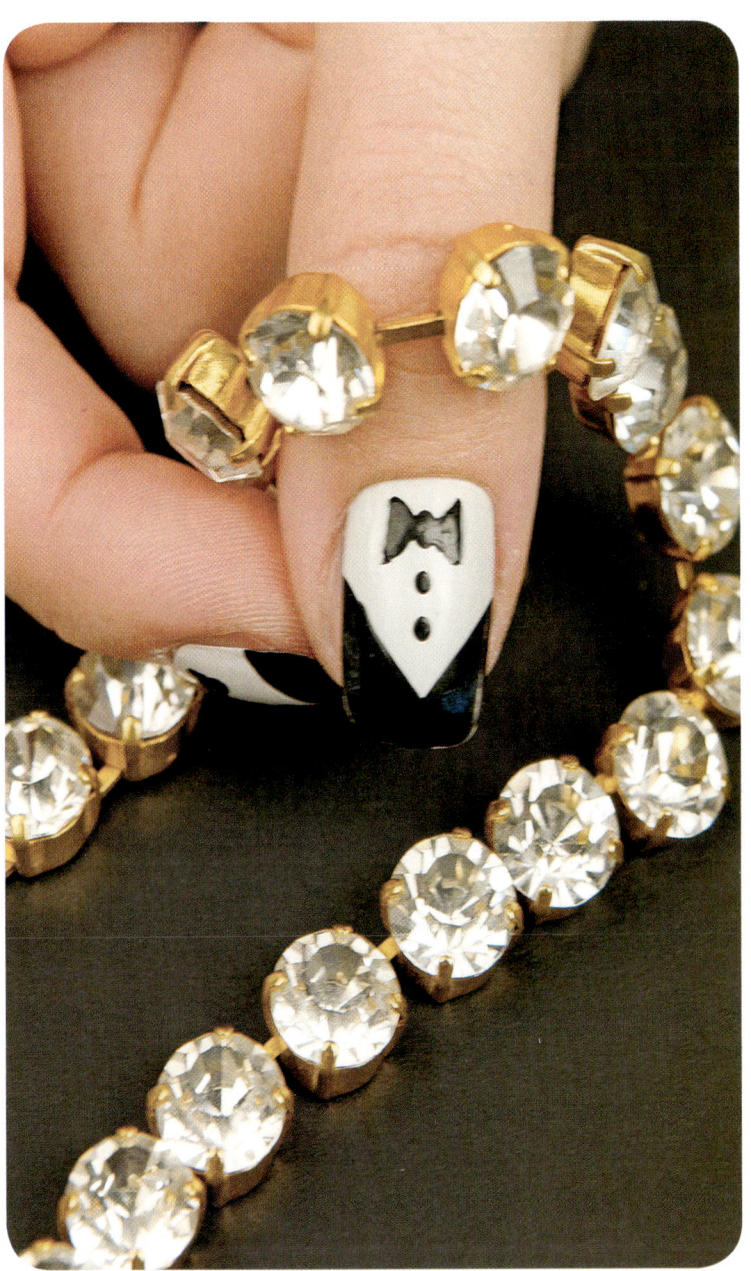

Difficulty ✽✽✽

# MEOW!
## Fur and claws

fine brush and dotter | base coat | white, black, green, and pink nail polish | | top coat

1. Apply a base coat to the nails and, once dry, apply two coats of white nail polish. Let dry.

2. For the paw prints: with the dotter, dipped in black nail polish, make a circle with three dots above it for the toe print.

3. For the cat: with the brush dipped in black nail polish, draw the outline of the cat. With the tip of the brush, dipped in pink, draw the nose and the inside of the ears. With the dotter dipped in the green, make the eyes, and with the brush and black polish make the pupils. Three fine gray stripes on the sides of the nose will be the whiskers.

4. Finish with an application of top coat.

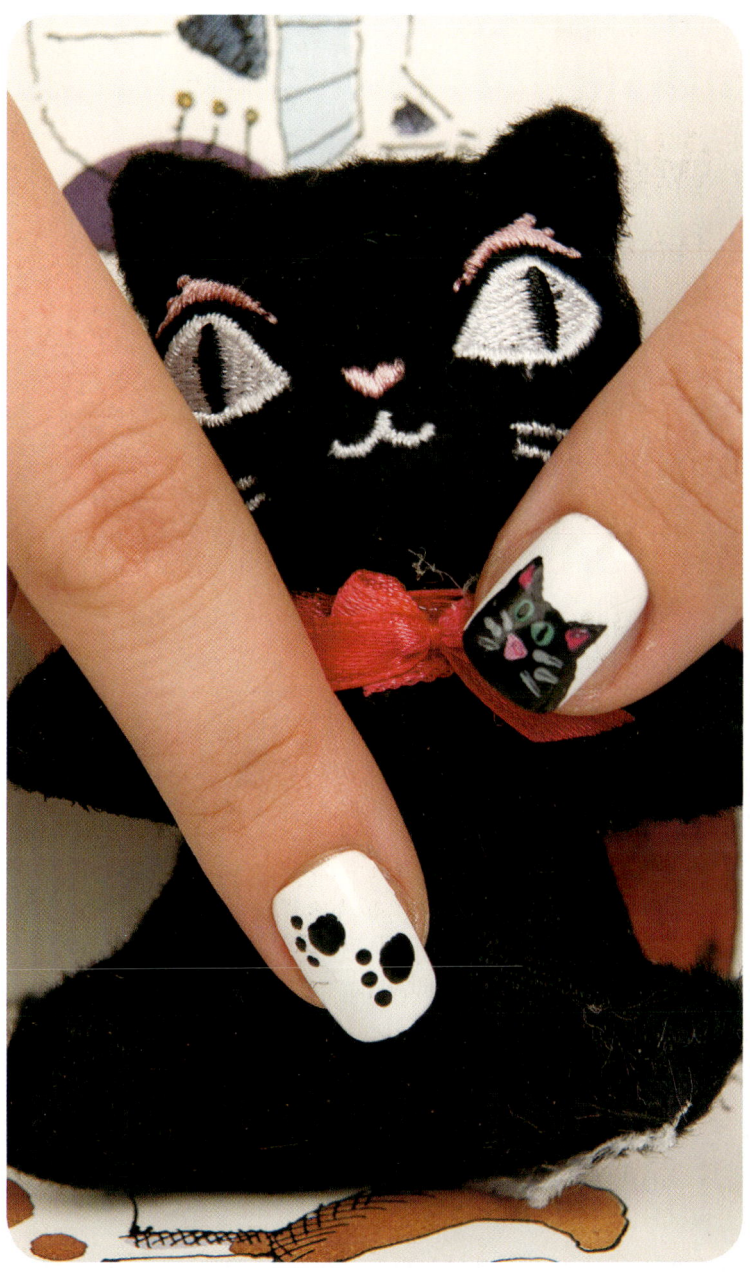

Difficulty ✸

# Goth
*Soul rebel*

tweezers / base coat / brightly colored nail polish / skull nail tattoos / top coat

1. Apply the base coat and let dry.
2. Select a nail polish with a strong color that contrasts with the color of the skull nail tattoo, and apply it twice.
3. Take a skull nail tattoo and apply it gently with tweezers, to avoid damaging the nail polish.
4. When the tattoo has adhered perfectly, apply the top coat.

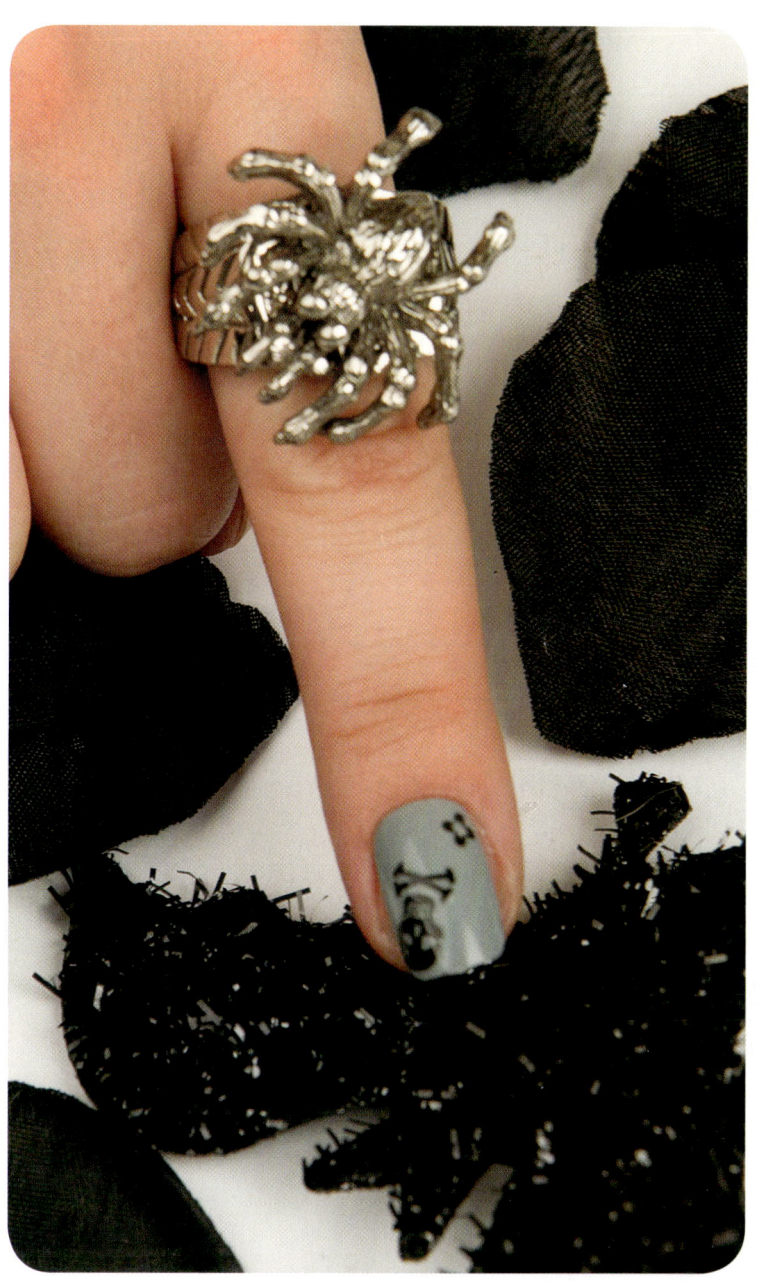

Difficulty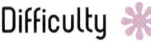

# It's springtime
## Flight of the butterflies

tweezers | base coat | brightly colored nail polish of your choice | butterfly and flower nail tattoos, rhinestones | top coat

1. Apply the base coat and let dry.
2. Choose a nail polish color that matches the nail tattoos and apply it twice over the base coat.
3. Take the nail tattoos and position them on the nail, sealing them with the top coat.
4. Repeat the process on all nails, alternating the decorations.

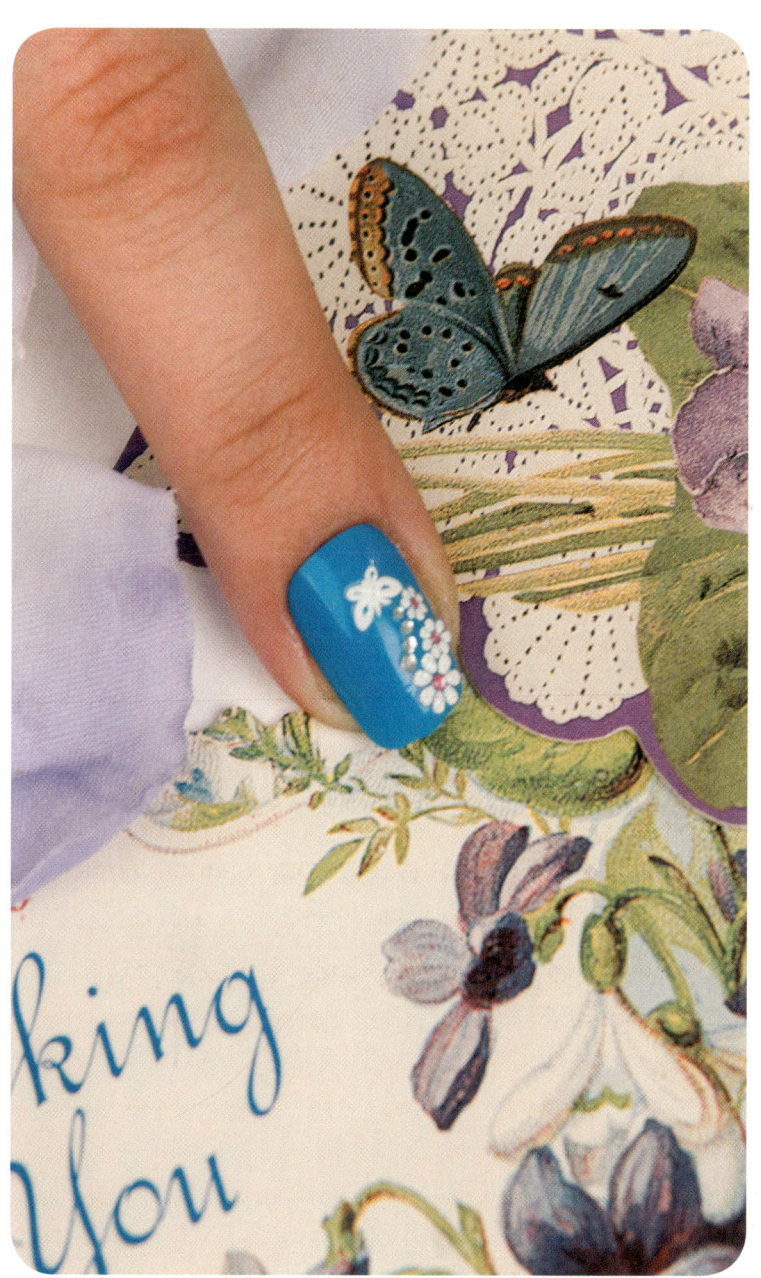

Difficulty ✸

# Romantic
## *For beautiful dreamers*

fine brush and dotter | base coat | brightly colored nail polish of your choice | nail tattoos with rhinestones or flowers | top coat

1. Apply the base coat and let dry.

2. Apply two coats of the nail polish of your choice; it is important that it contrasts with the color of the nail tattoo you have chosen.

3. Take the tattoos and, one by one, apply them gently onto your painted nails.

4. Make them adhere well and seal them with an application of top coat. Repeat this process on all the nails.

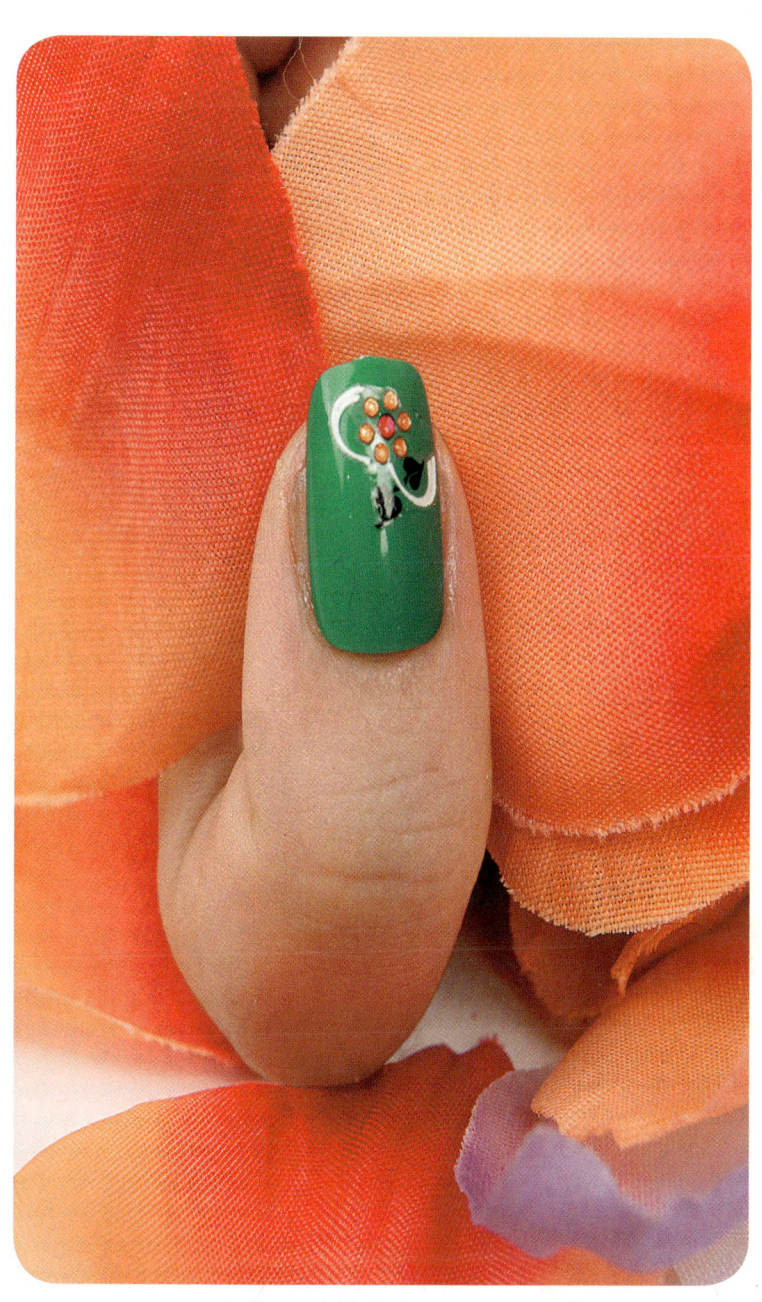